The Heart and Soul of Caregiving

Jacqueline Jennifer

This is a work of fiction. Names, characters, places, and incidents are the products of the author's imagination or are used fictiously. Any resemblance to actual events, locales or persons, living or dead, is entirely coincidental.

The Heart and Soul of Caregiving

Copyright ©2017 Jacqueline Jennifer

All Rights Reserved.

ISBN-13: 978-1543152913
ISBN-10: 1543152910

Library of Congress Control Number: 2017902484

CONTACT THE AUTHOR AT:

JOONJACKBOOKS@GMAIL.COM

PRAISE FOR
THE HEART AND SOUL OF CAREGIVING

"Success in any occupation can be defined in many ways. *The Heart and Soul of Caregiving* offers the honest and pure tenets of this admirable profession in a very thorough and comprehensive manner. The author speaks with clarity, heart and honesty. Using entertaining real life stories, this book defines the essential role of a caregiver."
~ *Dr. Daisy Quiblat, Medical Doctor*

"I have seen many stories described as heartwarming. I am 90 years old and this story is the first where I have felt the warmth."
~ *Robert E. Margolies, Retired Engineer*

"Do you ever wonder who will be at your side when you take your last breath? If your family is lucky, healthcare worker Jacqueline Jennifer will be among them and this moving personal testimony will tell you why."
~ *John Bonaduce, Musical Director*

Praise for
The Heart and Soul of Caregiving

"I quote the author, *Not everyone in their career has this kind of opportunity to make a difference in someone's life.* The author describes this experience so eloquently. Bittersweet, but oh so worth it."

~ *Evangeline Reid, Caregiver*

"*The Heart and Soul of Caregiving* is truly heartwarming. Quality caregiving is a memorable experience that will last a lifetime."

~ *Aimee Del Campo, Registered Nurse*

"*The Heart and Soul of Caregiving* is a book that every caregiver should read. As an RN and having a daughter that runs a senior center, I realize how critical it is to have a caregiver that is not judgmental, but rather loving, caring and respectful. Having seen the author in action, she really does live all the wonderful traits that she thinks a caregiver should possess. Her clients are lucky to have her. If I ever need a caregiver, this book is a must read."

~ *Betty Odello, Registered Nurse*

The Heart and Soul of Caregiving

DEDICATION

This life is filled with so many challenges and uncertainties and I am just so blessed to always have my family by my side, through thick and thin.

To my husband, who is my *perfect* half. I cannot imagine how my life would have been, or will be, without him to share it with. This makes me so lucky! Thank you for loving me and making me feel so special. You are my best friend.

To our three boys, our angels, the love of our lives and the best gift that God gave us. Thank you for being so great and loving. You are always our joy and laughter.

To our moms and aunts who were always there to guide us throughout our lives. Thank you for your love and patience, and for being our inspirations.

Jacqueline Jennifer

The love you all showed us growing up is the foundation that molded me to be the person that I am now.

To our dads, who we lost early in life, who I know are looking down upon us from Heaven.

To our brothers and sisters and our whole family that makes living more meaningful and exciting. For me, without love and family, life wouldn't be as interesting. (And most especially the drama that goes with it!)

To my friends, the families of Peter, Ann and Eileen, who have been our inspiration. They taught me the beauty of love within the family. Nothing is perfect and everyone is different but the love they shared among each other opened my eyes to the beauty and greatness of relationships. I am grateful for their unconditional and overwhelming

The Heart and Soul of Caregiving

love and support, and for opening their hearts and homes to us, most especially during those years when we were away from our families.

To Eileen, my idol, my friend. Like you, I want to wear purple when I grow old. You are a rock star!

To Anne, for all the kisses and the hugs and the *I love you's* you gave me each day we were together. You made me feel so loved, like a mother. And thank you for laughing at my jokes all the time!

To Peter, our rock. You calmed down our worries and comforted us with your wisdom. You always listened and showered me with praises and affection. When things were rough and uncertain, you never failed to assure us that everything will be okay. You were always right. Thank you for sharing how you raised your boys. They are all great! You

Jacqueline Jennifer

are our inspiration in raising our family. Now that you're gone, whenever I find myself unsure and confused, I go back to how you would have talked to me, *that everything will be okay.* And it will be. And for sure, it will.

To Laurie, Skip and Paul, who helped me start my own caregiving business. Thank you for believing in me and always supporting me and my family. You are our mentors and our great friends. Thank you for all your love and faith in us. You have touched our lives in the most special way. Forever, we are grateful.

To our Angel Care Team, my friends, my caregivers who are out there each day sharing their love and their hearts with our clients, I thank you all. I am always humbled by your patience, kindness and unconditional love that you

The Heart and Soul of Caregiving

give our patients. I know how challenging it is and at the same time so rewarding. Having the privilege of having you all on my team makes me feel so lucky and proud. You are great warriors, literally and genuinely our Angels.

To God, for allowing me to discover this great opportunity to be a part of other people's lives and have the privilege of making a difference. It is such an honor and a blessing.

This book is dedicated most especially to the memory of Eileen, Peter and Ann, and the greatness of their families whom we had the privilege and honor of knowing. We can never be grateful enough.

~ Jacqueline Jennifer

The Heart and Soul of Caregiving

In life, there are jobs, professions, vocations and callings. Some of us stumble upon a job. An interest leads one to a profession. A belief or suitability directs someone to their vocation. A calling is a strong urge or an inner drive to provide a service or a task. Successful caregivers are answering their calling.

A firefighter must go to school to learn the chemical composition of a fire, the specifics of hazardous materials and the many structural elements of a building. School will not teach courage, another job requirement. Courage is an element the firefighter was born with, a value that has been tested throughout his or her life. Courage lies in their hearts and souls.

The skills with which *to give care* are many. There are practical skills for efficient problem solving; these can be learned. Most of the successful caregiver's attributes are inherent, innate and inborn. Patience. Joy. Insight into human nature. Awareness and respect for the process of life. A desire to please, unselfishly. It takes a very special person to turn pain and fear into comfort and ease.

The American population is aging, rapidly. People are living much lon-

The Heart and Soul of Caregiving

ger than ever before. Senior citizens are a growing population. Who will take care of them? Caregiving is intensely personal. What does the job entail? Who can one trust?

Following are just several stories out of hundreds that define a caregiver. Early in my career, my eyes were wide open to the new profession. This is when I saw and learned the most. Details of each day, aspects of personalities and so many needs offer an insight into the heart and soul of a caregiver.

Eileen

When I started to take a caregiving job, I had no clue what to expect or do. I grew up with helpers and nannies around me and was never taught the basic tasks of cleaning and cooking. Even my kids had their own nannies. However, I thought, I had a Management Degree and business background. How hard could it be? I needed a job to support my family and whatever it takes I will do it.

Jacqueline Jennifer

So with that boost of confidence and positive attitude, I met with my client Eileen. Right there and then, she sized me up from head to toe. I bet she was thinking, "This girl looks clueless as a deer in headlights. How on earth can she help me?" I stared back at her thinking...oh God, she can smell my fear! I never felt so scared in my life! I thought, this is something I didn't think through and there was no way out. I kept telling myself, be brave, I can do it, she's just another person, I will make it out alive! Her daughter broke the ice by introducing herself and her mother. She showed me the medications that her mom needed and she gave me a tour of their house.

First Day

Eileen told me everything I needed to do, which was helpful. My patient was in pain due to a hip fracture and she depended a lot on pain medications. She moved around with a walker but would ask me to bring her stuff when she was sitting down in her TV room. She was so nice but she could be so feisty at the same time because she was in such pain. I felt for her and understood her condition, but no amount of patience and care could shield my feelings from getting hurt when I got snapped at. I tried to be more patient and understanding and did my best in doing my job diligently. I had to make it work.

At the end of the day, I walked to the bus.

Back then, I had no car. I waited at the bus stop for thirty minutes and I cried. I had a big pity party all the way home! I thought, *Wow, I've never had to serve anyone in my life*. I really did not mind it at all, but that experience made me feel so insulted and hurt and so demeaning! I felt so down, defeated and angry, at my situation. No amount of Management Skills could help me out this time. So much for positive thinking.

The Second Day

Eileen asked me to wash the rags I used to clean the house. I happily did it in the sink and used Ajax as soap. Eileen went ballistic and asked me what in the world was I doing with the Ajax. I proudly replied, "I'm washing the rags." She told me I couldn't do that because Ajax is for scouring the sink or tiles and not to be used as a soap.

I stood my ground and argued with her saying, *"But this is soap, right?"*

Jacqueline Jennifer

Eileen just laughed. She couldn't get over it. She said, "Oh, I get it now.... You don't know anything about cleaning!"

I felt ashamed. My pride was hurt. But I was sort of glad though, as she was in good spirits and found it amusing.

So we sat down, had coffee and I told her all about my inexperience with household chores. I explained to her how my parents brought up me and my siblings (all five of us) with helpers so they could both work. They were both doing very well with their jobs. They were both very good providers. In the Philippines, wages are just a fraction of what it cost here in the United States. Providing us with helpers gave them peace of mind while leaving us home by ourselves. Because of that kind of upbringing, we

The Heart and Soul of Caregiving

lived a sheltered life and never had to do any chores. I never even had to make my own bed or clean my own room, not because I didn't want to, but because I never had to. I was honest about it and told her I was willing to learn.

She said, "Well, we need to educate you!" She taught me the different safe and old-fashioned style of cleaning products. I never imagined that vinegar could be used for cleaning. I had never pondered how things should be done. I was amazed at how organized and thorough she was. And as promised, I was the perfect student. I learned so much from her and I was grateful for that. Since then, I did things exactly as she wanted them done.

On my way home, walking to Sunset Boulevard, I realized that life is not

Jacqueline Jennifer

as bad as it seemed. Things get better and I was thankful for a productive day.

Things got better. I knew where things were, which made it less frustrating for Eileen when she needed something. She invited me to watch her soap opera *As the World Turns*. I made her tea in the English way, just as she liked it.

Things were better, until one day, her friend Nick came to visit and have coffee with her. I helped prepare and serve their beverages. All of a sudden, Eileen snapped at me because I did not use the right plate to serve the cookies.

I felt embarrassed and humiliated in front of her friend. I had to hold back the tears that were about to fall. I excused myself and went in the backyard where the laundry was and stayed there for a while.

The Heart and Soul of Caregiving

I knew I had to be patient because she didn't mean to be nasty or rude. She was in pain and had the tendency to be grouchy. I kept telling myself this while doing the laundry. Suddenly, Nick came after me and apologized for Eileen. He explained that she's not her usual self. I told him I very much understood. But I got more embarrassed, because the tears just poured like crazy. I was overwhelmed with that negative experience and I got so emotional. I was not upset or mad. I totally felt for Eileen, but I guess I couldn't stop myself from feeling hurt.

So again, I walked home in tears. I was feeling sorry for myself, asking *Why do I have to do this job?* But I knew why. I needed a job to survive. I had to stop whining and acting like a baby. I had to start to make things work.

I thought, *This should be so easy.* I just needed to think how to make it work. It's not like I had a choice. So on the way home, I stopped crying and I started to think how I could be not only a good caregiver for Eileen, but also the best she will ever have. Maybe my Management and Business skills won't be useless after all!

First Step: Attitude Change

I needed a whole new mindset and perspective. I love and respect myself because I am a good person and I have earned a good education. If I degrade myself, how can other people respect me? I was doing a very significant job and I just needed to see how important my role was in my patient's life. It was an opportunity to do well and be good at it.

Jacqueline Jennifer

Not everyone in their own career field has this kind of opportunity to make a difference in someone else's life, right? It could be a life changing career choice for me, so I had to be very professional about it and take it seriously.

Having that now in mind, I felt completely empowered and driven. I was very excited.

Then the next big question hit. *How?* What's the Second Step? And I quote Eileen's favorite expression, "It ain't easy, Miggie!"

Second Step

It didn't come easy.

There was no manual for it.

I just did my job in the most efficient way possible. I did the right thing. I followed the routine that Eileen wanted. She had a very structured and organized way of living.

Then one day, and I quote her again by saying, "I had a brainwave!" She kept complaining about her disorganized laundry room; it has been that way

Jacqueline Jennifer

for years. It drove her crazy just thinking about it since she has never been so disorganized in all her life. So I thought, *Why not make a project out of it?*

I told her one morning, "Let's go in the back. You can sit in the garden chair and supervise how you want me to clean out and organize the laundry room." That day, we tackled the big project. I brought all the stuff out to the garden and I cleaned the whole room. We threw away a lot of stuff. At the end of the day, we both were worn out but it made her extremely happy.

After the big job she called all her friends. Her daughter told everyone how amazing I was. She said that the laundry room was so clean and organized, they could have a tea party in it!

The Heart and Soul of Caregiving

The praise was really nothing compared to the amount of joy I felt. It was the most awesome and rewarding feeling I have ever had in my life. I thought, *What a huge difference a small amount of good work and gesture can make. If we can all go the extra mile to make a person feel happy or just even smile, it really goes a long way.*

I may not have had Eileen at Hello... but I had her when I organized her laundry room!

Going the Extra Mile

It was a great feeling knowing that I made her day. At least for that day I did.

One thing I have learned through the years in caring for the elderly is to take things one day at a time.

My lack of domestic skills, which I mastered through the years with Eileen's expert coaching, was forgiven, as my other skills, such as my knowledge in computers and technology, were much

Jacqueline Jennifer

needed. That is one area where she had no knowledge and somehow, I gained her respect by doing things for her that she cannot do herself. One example was when I scanned her photos and made copies for her to give to her friends. She thought that was amazing. I fixed her remote when she accidentally pushed the wrong buttons. I changed her bulbs and I fixed her fax. I used my Management skills by helping with her correspondence and filing, dealing with her doctors, setting up a workable system for her healthcare needs. Since then, I have focused on things that made her happy, on a day-to-day basis. I think that after I organized her laundry room, there was nothing I could do was wrong...Ha-ha. But seriously, I had a clear mindset to do my best to make her life easier and

The Heart and Soul of Caregiving

happier. We laughed and cried together, we even got pissed at the same things. We actually took care of each other and learned a lot from each other.

Focus on What is Important

Every person is different. We just need to focus on what that person values and what makes that person happy. It's a guide that has worked for me during the eight years we were together. She passed recently and I never thought I could cry for somebody that much. Eileen always told me how similar we were. Our birthdays are a day apart. We're both Aquarians. For some reason, we think alike and we *are* alike, in so many ways. It was a

Jacqueline Jennifer

beautiful relationship, for we had that strong connection. She was like a sister, a best friend, a mother...all in one. She told me we were like two peas in a pod, soulmates. We had a good run for eight years. I have great memories of fun, learning, and love.

No Crossing the Line

I loved her like family, but as a caregiver, I never crossed that line with her, or any client. It is a pitfall for some. They take advantage of the close relationships they develop with their clients, and fail to draw the line between personal and professional. I am a professional caregiver and I separate my job from personal issues. That way, I know that I will always do what's right. I also learned that by drawing that line

Jacqueline Jennifer

clearly, I gained her respect for being professional in my job. I loved Eileen as a friend and I respected her as a boss or client. I think that's one of the reasons why I became good and effective in my job, and why we had a lasting successful relationship. I can proudly say that I was the best caregiver she ever had.

My Personal Letter to Eileen

My Ever Dearest Eileen,

You are the most beautiful and graceful Dutch ballerina dancer I ever had the honor of meeting. You have an amazing spirit and are one of the most selfless people I have known. It was a great honor being a part of your life. I miss you terribly and it helps writing this book to honor you, and remember you. You were a bright light that shined upon me, dur-

Jacqueline Jennifer

ing those years of being far away from my family.

Who would have thought that our lives would cross and share beautiful memories together? You always thanked me for everything but you never realized how much you have helped me too. You took care of me in your own way by making me feel loved and important. I miss your leftover soup and your Dutch cookies that you gave me to nibble while I took the bus home. I recall the times you picked me up on Rexford when you were still strong enough to drive. Remember how we criticized that ugly looking big house under construction? You always insisted on picking me up from the bus stop and driving me back after work. I miss your cards every birthday, Mother's Day, Easter, Christmas and Valentines Day. I

The Heart and Soul of Caregiving

miss the stationery and cards you gave me that you got from the charities that drove you crazy each time they gave you small gifts and you felt compelled to give back. I miss when you called to check in and ask how my day was, or when you just wanted to bitch about someone who annoyed you that day. Every time I see tulips, I remember you. You influenced me to buy half and half from Trader Joe's that I use in my coffee once in a while.

Through the years, I never realized how huge a part you were in my life. I'm sorry I never told you that enough. I guess I always felt you would be around forever. I didn't even record your experiences during the war, when you were in Holland growing up. There are just too many unsaid words and things left undone. I can still hear your voice some-

Jacqueline Jennifer

times, because it is so familiar to me. I remember the times when you called and we both had a cocktail or wine and just laughed at silly things. I miss those days. You were always there for me and I thank you for that. Whenever I was upset about something and I told you about it, it was so funny how you were more upset than me! I ended up consoling you, instead of the other way around! That's why I tried not to tell you upsetting stories, because you would lose sleep over it. Like the one time when I had a fraudulent withdrawal from my bank account, you really went at it with me every day to make sure I got my money back. You got so majorly pissed, you even told all your friends about it. That is why I am missing you more now, because every time I have problems or exciting news, you are

The Heart and Soul of Caregiving

*no longer there to call. I miss you on the other end of the line. I miss coming to see you. You always greeted me with a sigh, saying, "Oh, it's only 10 a.m. and I am already exhausted!" It was so funny how you would let me know all the things you did over the weekend, because you felt guilty if you didn't do anything. It's funny because I was like that too! You would tell me, "It doesn't look like I did a lot, but I really did!" I think I started to act like you over the years. I'm glad I did, because you are so cool and **you rock!** I want to be like you when I grow old.*

I will forever value the overwhelming love that you shared with me.

Respectfully,
Jacqueline

Jacqueline Jennifer

What once started as an impossible scenario with Eileen turned out to be a wonderful and loving relationship. Eileen looked out for me like a mother hen. I was looking for additional work. A local boutique hotel wanted to hire me and Eileen totally discouraged the idea. She was afraid that some crazy guest could take advantage of me, given that there was no security in the building. I honestly had never even thought of that; I just couldn't afford to think of those things when I was so focused on earning extra income. The manager offered me a full time job to manage the hotel when she was away. It was a very tempting offer. It was more money and financial stability.

However, I couldn't leave Eileen, because I knew that was not the right thing for me to do. For someone who needed more income, money was the last thing on my mind and I decided to decline the hotel offer. Instead, I persistently begged Eileen to help me ask around among her friends in the neighborhood for a job. I had no car and commuting from one job to another was impractical, time wise. I let my worries go, did what I had to do, and put my faith in my decision to do what I thought was right. I hoped that I was right.

Power of the Mind

How amazing it is to focus on a goal and watch the opportunities come knocking in! After a few days, a friend of Eileen called and asked for help because a neighbor was suffering from Alzheimer's and the family needed a caregiver. Eileen mentioned that I was looking for an extra job and that I was available. I thought, "Wow, my prayers are answered." I just prayed and prayed and let go.

Jacqueline Jennifer

Weeks went by and finally I received a call from Paul, the son, and he discussed with me his mother's care needs. However, Peter, the father, was in complete denial. For him, a caregiver was totally out of the question because he believed that his wife was okay and that he could take good care of her. They had four sons and all siblings were clueless as to how they were going to convince their father to agree that their mom needed care.

First of all, in all honesty, that was the first time I had heard about Alzheimer's. I learned that their mom drove her car and got lost a few times. As days passed, she started knocking on neighbors' doors claiming she was lost. One time she was found sleeping under a parked truck at the side of the road.

The Heart and Soul of Caregiving

The neighbors called the police a couple of times, which pressured the sons to do something about the situation. They had meeting after meeting trying to figure out how to convince their dad. They always reached a dead end whenever they confronted their father because they knew there was no way they could make him agree.

So finally, after another phone call from Paul, we decided to meet at Eileen's house to discuss the situation. I can never forget that day. Eileen gave us some space; she let us talk at her kitchen table. Paul gave me the whole scenario and I felt his frustrations. Based on what he told me about his father, it reminded me of my own dad. He was so proud that he never admitted he needed help from anyone. I could relate to him and

Jacqueline Jennifer

suddenly I had a great idea, what Eileen called "a brain wave." The dad couldn't walk much because of a knee problem and he could no longer accompany his wife on a walk. I suggested we offer my help to go walking with Ann, the mom, so she will have her exercise.

    At least that was a good way of introducing myself to his dad. Before we got to talk, Eileen gave me an impression that Peter, the dad, was a difficult man. Maybe he was grumpy, which worried me a lot. When I asked son Paul about that, he said that his dad was a very gracious, nice man and I had nothing to worry about. I figured that Eileen had that cranky impression of Peter because he was a Republican. Eileen was a Democrat and they used to argue a lot in the past. How funny is that?!

The Heart and Soul of Caregiving

Paul drove with me to visit with his dad who was just a block away up the canyon. We went in, and when I saw Peter, sitting on his couch, smoking his pipe, I immediately fell in love with him. He was so much like my grandfather. And he was reading a book of Shakespeare! It brought me back in time when my grandfather would spend most of his waking hours reading Shakespeare, smoking a pipe and listening to classical music. It melted my heart. Indeed, he was very nice and sat with us at the dining table. He said it was a nice surprise to see his son Paul.

Then, I met Ann. She came to me and gave me her toothbrush. She was really confused, but her smile was sweet and childlike. Paul introduced us and told his dad that I will be coming by to accompany Ann on a walk everyday. His dad said it was a great idea.

That was it. Paul was speechless for a few seconds and decided to leave right away. He told his dad he needed to get back to his office. I think our visit only lasted five minutes. I guess he wanted to rush out because he was worried his dad might change his mind.

He offered to drive me home. As we got to his car, he just blurted out how happy he was. He felt like he had won the lottery! Now employed, I had this overwhelming feeling of relief and happiness. I felt so happy for him too! He was like a kid on Christmas Day with all the presents!

Although I was subconsciously reprimanding myself for getting into a situation that was way over my head, I

The Heart and Soul of Caregiving

was overcome with so much admiration for the love that I witnessed in this very extraordinary family. It was so touching and I knew that I would give everything to make it work. It was like a mission for me and it motivated me to help out their family. I felt so blessed to be a part of that beautiful family.

That night, after a glass of wine, contemplating all that happened that day, it suddenly hit me. I had no idea whatsoever how to handle the job that I just accepted, and this family was counting on me to help their mom! I did panic and hyperventilate. I talked myself into calming down. It was going to be okay. I kept repeating but it took awhile before I believed myself. What was I thinking?

After a deep, deep breath, I remembered the happiness and the hope

Jacqueline Jennifer

I brought to that family. How hard could it be, right? I prayed for strength and sanity and reflection. I came to realize that I could do it. Simply because, if it were my mother, I would do anything to take care of her. I just had to do what I had to do like a daughter would do for her mom. So that was my mindset. It worked for me.

That night, I started reading about Alzheimer's and learned that it was a degenerative disease. I felt so sad and sorry for Ann and for Peter and their sons. I knew it was going to be one of the biggest challenges in my life. I may have been lacking in experience, but I knew that my heart was ready for the job. And that was all I needed to make it work.

When I came to work the next day, I found Ann in bed, soaking wet, trying

The Heart and Soul of Caregiving

to get out of her clothes. She looked at me, helpless like a child. Luckily, she trusted me enough to help her out.

First Things First

When you are clueless to what you're doing, focus on the here and now. One step at a time. I thought, I knew what to do, take her to the bathroom, clean her up so she'll feel more comfortable, dress her up, then make breakfast.

We did that without any resistance at all. I was so happy I was able to help Ann get all cleaned up. That was a lucky break. Peter made breakfast, which was so sweet. Ann finished her food and took

Jacqueline Jennifer

her medicines diligently. Then we started walking.

Okay, I need to do some explaining. I know most people in LA are exceptionally fit and into physical fitness, yoga and Pilates, but I had to walk thirty-seven minutes from Sunset before I even began work. We cannot forget that I have to walk thirty-seven minutes back to the bus stop in the evening. So I think my getting tired walking up and down the street was pretty much valid. The thing was, Ann was a hiker. She hiked up mountains with her husband and kids when they were growing up. She was more fit than I have ever been in my lifetime. It was embarrassing to admit that.

On top of it, since she had Alzheimer's, the hiker forgot that we had

The Heart and Soul of Caregiving

already gone for a walk. Finally, after the tenth long march, I talked her out of another. I told her she was already tired. In truth, I was the one who was tired and worn out. I never wanted to admit that to myself. Even now, remembering it, makes me embarrassed.

Our scenario was, after walking up the long street and back, we would march into the house and sit on the couch. I would make a big sigh of relief. Then, after a heartbeat, she would turn to me and say, "Let's go for a walk!"

I was like, "Huh?"

Then she smiled, taunting me. How could I say "No"? After a few days of the same dilemma, I tried to evaluate my attitude. I couldn't afford getting upset about a situation that I had no control of. Exercise was good. Agitating

Jacqueline Jennifer

Ann was not good. So instead of expecting her to throw pity on me, I had to face the fact that she will never back down. Therefore, I had to accept that we were going to take a walk fifteen to twenty times a day.

This is part of the job and the end of the story.

Love... Love... Love...

I walked in the house one morning slowly closing the door behind me and as I tiptoed to the bedroom to check on Ann and Peter. I heard them talking in the bathroom which was at the end of the hallway. I was taken aback when I saw Peter helping Ann change her diaper. After she got dressed, Peter combed her hair. I watched them both with admiration for their love. It was a very beautiful thing to witness and right then

Jacqueline Jennifer

I understood why Peter was against having a caregiver for his wife; he wanted to be able to take care of her.

Ann had Alzheimer's and forgot all the names of her family members except Peter's. She called him by name and looked at him with so much love. It was amazing to witness such powerful emotions.

They usually sat across from each other at the dining room table. Every so often they would look at each other, smile and throw kisses. Sometimes Ann would walk to his side and cuddle beside him. She may have forgotten a great deal but the love she felt for Peter was the very thing she never forgot. He was the only joy she had each day, from the moment she woke up to the time she went to bed. Her whole life revolved around

The Heart and Soul of Caregiving

Peter. He was her reason to live. It was truly amazing to have been a witness to such a beautiful love story.

The Kids

My feelings for Ann and Peter's children were kind of funny and strange at the same time. They had four amazing sons, who were of course all grown up, but since I was taking care of their parents and having my own boys as well, I saw them as Peter saw "his boys," like they were kids.

Peter always told me wonderful stories about them growing up. How they traveled all over the United States and other countries. He was so proud that he and his boys climbed so many mountains. Ann would carry them on her shoulder when they were little. Ann even kept a log of their vacations. She was mighty efficient in her journals; all her logs were neatly typewritten. I wonder where she got the time to be organized on top of taking care of four boys!

I was a witness to the love they shared as a family. I saw how the sons struggled in the beginning about the care for their parents and each other's contribution. Of course they had many disagreements, but one thing was very clear: they all shared the same love and respect for their mom and dad. I cannot say one loved them more than the other. I believe that they coped differently. Ev-

The Heart and Soul of Caregiving

eryone had his own unique role. It was simply amazing to be a part of that experience.

Respect

I took it upon myself to call "the boys" whenever Peter wanted to talk or to remind them to visit. I also assumed the role of the General Manager of the house, by making sure all appointments were met, supplies were bought and chores were done.

However, I needed a day or two off. Peter did not want to have anyone else in the house but me. While this was completely understandable, it created an-

Jacqueline Jennifer

other dilemma for his boys. Again, they discussed how they could convince their dad to find a substitute. Sometimes they casually asked Peter during a conversation and Peter would casually disagree with them. What really touched me was their manner and attitude in dealing with their dad.

One morning before breakfast, Skip and Paul came by to visit unannounced, which surprised Peter and I. Skip and Paul asked their dad to join them for a discussion. With his pipe in hand, Peter got up and moved to the head of the dining room table. Each son took a side. Asked to join, I felt kind of awkward because I knew that they would be trying to convince their dad to allow another caregiver to relieve me. It was so funny because they approached him in

The Heart and Soul of Caregiving

a very formal and business-like manner. On a yellow legal pad, Skip wrote down all the advantages and disadvantages of having help in the house. Peter nodded the entire time as each son made his case. Peter thanked them for coming and politely said that he does not agree with what they were saying. He then excused himself and left the room. Right after he left, Skip and Paul sighed with frustration and resignation. I laughed because I could not contain myself. I told them that they were both CEOs of their own big companies yet they couldn't win a case against their father. It was really a heart-warming experience to see and feel their love and respect for their dad. The boys never raised their voices or got upset when they did not get what they wanted. Mostly, they felt frustrated but

Jacqueline Jennifer

ultimately they let their dad make all the final decisions. Honestly, that was a first for me. I come from a big family and we always ended up shouting at each other with doors banging and eyes rolling. In the end, Peter agreed that they would only need additional care if I were to be gone for more than four days in a row.

Not long after, clever son Paul asked me if I would take a week long, all expenses paid vacation to Las Vegas so they could hire a substitute. They even gave me money to see a show! What a treat! Win-Win!

INTERESTING WALKS WITH ANN

Alzheimer's is a very challenging disease for the patient, the family and the caregivers. Ann was such an amazing lady and I knew that even though I never got the privilege of knowing her before she developed her disease, I could tell that she was a great lady. She was graceful in so many ways. She was a great mother and she was a very loving wife. As clueless as I was when I started to take care of Ann, I created a list of long

Jacqueline Jennifer

and short-term goals. The long-term goals were all about health, well-being and a very good quality of life. The short-term goals were about achieving success in our daily routines such as taking all her pills, having her eat delicious and nutritious food and personal hygiene. The most important goal I set for myself each day was to make her laugh or to make her feel happy and comforted. I was amazed at how she would laugh at my corny jokes and listen to my boring stories with great interest. She made me laugh many times and often told me she loved me. She was the one person in my life who said "I love you" the most; she would repeat it every minute of every day. I never got tired of hearing it. I told her I loved her as well.

I felt her love for me as a moth-

The Heart and Soul of Caregiving

er loves a child. It was strange, but that was how I truly felt. She made me feel loved in her own special way. I remember the times when she would kiss my hand. Sometimes she would bite it instead of kissing it! I would get startled and she would look at me mischievously as though she knew that it would make me laugh every time. I always gave her warm hugs and kisses. It was so easy to love her.

I asked myself at the end of each day, "Did Ann have a good quality of life? Did she go to bed feeling loved and comforted? Did she have a productive day?"

A caregiver's job is always one day at a time. Although she had Alzheimer's and had lost most of her memory, Ann was highly intuitive. She could sense if

Jacqueline Jennifer

she was loved. Because of the bond that we shared, she would always recognize me, even after a few days apart. She never remembered my name, but every time she saw me, she had that look of love and familiarity.

I remember once during a day off, I decided to pay them a visit to see how the new caregiver was working out. The moment Ann saw me, she ran towards me like a little kid. The caregiver held her arm to slow her down. Ann shoved her away and said, "Leave me alone!" It was surprising to see that reaction. I wondered why Ann was reacting that way towards her. Ann grabbed my hand and pleadingly asked me if I would take her for a walk. As we strolled the neighborhood, I felt how happy she was to see me. Maybe this other caregiver was

The Heart and Soul of Caregiving

not connecting with her as much as she should?

For me, caregiving is not only about the basic care. It is the whole lifestyle, with the goal of giving and creating happiness and compassion. Connecting with a patient is just as important as providing meals, medications and personal hygiene. This is my personal opinion based upon my experiences. Ann was like a child who needed someone to guide her, to comfort her, to embrace her and to love her. Each day was always a new beginning, as memories are lost. What remains is the love and comfort that she felt from her family and those around her.

Every Tuesday

Peter would always play badminton every Tuesday with his son Paul. It has been their tradition for more than twenty years. Most times, Ann and I would stay home and wait for them to get back. They left at 6 P.M. and would return two hours later.

One Tuesday was the exception. Paul arrived with a balloon and cake! I was surprised to learn that Peter asked Paul to bring a cake and balloons for *my*

Jacqueline Jennifer

birthday! It was so sweet because I did not know about it; they had planned the celebration behind my back. I was so touched. I felt so loved and so special. They sang Happy Birthday and made me blow out the candles! That was really precious. They toasted me with a glass of wine. When I looked at Ann, her whole face was covered with chocolate cake! She smiled like a little kid. Awww. I miss her so much.

Paul drove me home as he usually did every Tuesday. We would often share stories on the short drive home. We did not agree most of the time, but we always ended up laughing. He was such a great friend, a wonderful son and an amazing person. I was so lucky to have met him. I enjoyed those times; they are all great memories.

Every Thursday

Right from the airport, Skip the eldest son and his wife Laurie would come and visit Peter and Ann. It was such joy to see Peter enjoying the fun conversations with Laurie and Skip and how much they appreciated one another. Skip would always start his conversations by telling him what was new. He would tell his dad interesting stories about his work and travels. Peter was so involved, listening to his son while smoking a pipe and

Jacqueline Jennifer

drinking his hot chocolate. I was always happy to see Peter retire at night with a smile on his face, happy and content after a great day.

Every Saturday

Brian came religiously every Saturday to his parents' house and did all the repairs needed. Whether it was the sink, which was always problematic, or a loose tile, or the maintenance of the car, it was Brian who got the job done.

I think most, if not all, elderly people have a hard time giving up their driver's license. Driving a car is the last bit of independence and mobility that they can cling to. Without the ability to

Jacqueline Jennifer

drive their own car, a senior feels like they are trapped and can no longer function. The elderly don't want to be told what they can or cannot do. I think it's proper to give our seniors the respect and dignity that they deserve. But I also believe that the family should be united in helping out their parents and do whatever is necessary for their parents', and other people's, safety and well-being.

That day came to Peter rather dramatically. My husband, who often drove Peter on his errands, took him to the DMV in order to renew his driver's license. Peter passed his written test and they automatically renewed his license! My husband carefully informed the DMV that the family felt that their father should not be driving anymore, so the department gave Peter a California

The Heart and Soul of Caregiving

Identification Card instead. Unfortunately, it looked very much like a Driver's License. We could never convince Peter that he did not have a license. It was not an argument that we could ever win.

Driving was no longer one of Peter's best skills. My husband would tell me how Peter would run down people in the supermarket aisle while driving one of those motorized carts. He even hit my husband a few times; he told me it was very, very painful.

The last time Peter drove his car, he got into an accident on Sunset and Beverly Drive. He claimed it was not his fault. I was just thankful that he got home in one piece, unharmed. He was shaking very badly. I guess that was his reality check. I bet all the neighbors were

Jacqueline Jennifer

relieved. They would always give Peter a five to ten minute head start whenever they saw him pull out of his driveway.

Brian, his brothers and I put our heads together to develop a strategy. We deflated the tires of Peter's car, so he would not be able to use it. The move was pretty sneaky, but we felt it was necessary for everyone's safety. It actually turned out pretty well!

Surprise Sundays

Tim the youngest among the brothers would surprise us mostly on Sundays for a visit with a new date. Peter was a ladies' man and he loved chatting with them. At some point I stopped memorizing their names because he introduced different women every few weeks. It was actually fun and entertaining for us because Peter and I would grade them after they left from 1 to 10. I suggested having a log book so we know who's who.

Jacqueline Jennifer

I was just kidding of course! They were all very nice and Peter always enjoyed a good conversation with the ladies. Peter was lucky to have his children visit him often, it really was always the highlight of his days each time he saw his boys. They were lucky too for having a great dad who was so proud of all of them. He raised them well.

The Respect and Responsibility of Raising Elderly Parents

This family showed me the real meaning of love and respect for parents. I admire them with all my heart and I pray that my own boys will treat my husband and I the same way when they grow up. I noticed that children of the elderly patients whom I was caring for had mostly the same two issues. 1) Convincing their parents to have a caregiver and 2) convincing them to give up driving. I believe I remember one of them saying

Jacqueline Jennifer

"Over my dead body!!" I bet it was feisty Eileen…

One thing I realized and the family probably did too, was that you can never win an argument with your parents, most especially if they have been independent all their lives. Some would probably appreciate their kid's concern for them, but the ones I cared for thought otherwise and sometimes they were vocal about it. I remember Peter walked out of the door with his car keys and when he noticed that his tires were flat, he called the roadside assistance company to fix it. They came the next morning and inflated the tires. The guy asked, "Why are the tires deflated?" Of course, I kept quiet.

The thing is, most children love their parents and respect what they want

The Heart and Soul of Caregiving

in life, but I think we all need to look at the bigger picture. We all have a moral and social responsibility towards our parents and other people. If we think that our parents could get killed driving or cause harm to other people, we need to stop it. If the children are having a hard time convincing them, their doctors can help discuss the issue with our parents. It is easier said than done, but voicing out our concerns could make a huge difference, rather than brushing the issue aside.

I remember Eileen being upset about her daughter's "bright idea" that she should not drive anymore and take the cab instead. She ranted about it for days. I lovingly reminded her that her daughter has only one mother, whom she loved the most in her entire life. She

Jacqueline Jennifer

doesn't want to lose her. Eileen's driving worries her daughter and I understand how hard it is for Eileen to give it up, but there are more pros than cons if she decides to stop driving.

1. Eileen does not worry when pulling her car out of the driveway. Oh my goodness! Do you know that she would roll down the passenger window so she could hear if there's a car approaching. She can't see anything from her driveway. It's a blind curve, approaching her house. For some divine reason, she always managed to drive out and maneuver without any entanglements. But that canyon road is always an accident waiting to happen! When her muffler hit the pavement, she knew that she had turned the right way. It sounds crazy but I as-

sure you, it was super scary when I was the one sitting in the passenger seat!

2. Parking will never be an issue when taking a taxicab. She can be dropped off wherever she wants to go and get picked up. Very easy!

Eileen was really good at parking; I give her that. I went with her one time to the doctor's office and we had to park in one of those narrow garages. Her car was a huge, wide Buick sedan. I honestly don't know how she managed to park so perfectly in those tiny slots. She was so proud, every time I praised her parking skills.

3. It's more cost-effective to take a cab because she doesn't have to buy gasoline and pay for maintenance. Plus, ev-

erything she might need is conveniently close in Beverly Hills. It is not that expensive considering the comfort, practicality and safety. She deserved it.

4. Peace of mind for her daughter. This is one of the most important reasons why Eileen should give up driving.

5. She can still keep her independence and freedom because she can go whenever and wherever she wanted. She could afford it. There are many cab companies out there, 24/7.

When I started working for Ann and Peter, I took a cab to work once in a while. I got to know some really nice drivers and I kept their contact information so I could call them when I needed them. Sometimes I would set a schedule

The Heart and Soul of Caregiving

in advance. That way, I am sure I won't get stuck with rude and mean drivers. I told Eileen I could arrange the same for her. I had a long list of very nice drivers on my phone.

6. "You still have your license," I told her, "and you still have your car sitting in the garage.

"You still have the power to drive if you really wanted to. You have not lost it. You are just making smart decisions for yourself because you want to be safe and responsible." I think that did it.

She stopped driving and her daughter arranged with one of her friends to drive Eileen. It worked out very well. Eileen still made a lot of sarcastic remarks, but I believe she knew that her daughter was right.

Giving Back

One of the challenges I had to face was how to make life a lot easier for this family. The sons were all busy. They had their own families to take care of. How could I give care to them? I then decided that there should be an overall goal, which was to make sure that everything was taken care of so that the sons won't have to worry about anything with regards to their parents.

Jacqueline Jennifer

The ultimate goal was for the sons to enjoy their visits with their mom and dad. They would have a peace of mind knowing that their parents are okay at all times. I decided to take charge of everything. I reported to them with solutions to all of their problems and concerns. I did most of the thinking and came up with ideas and solutions. I wanted to give them the gift of peace of mind and worry-free and fun visits with their mom and dad. It was the least I could do for them.

I thought of myself as one of the luckiest people in the world. I never imagined how rewarding caregiving was. It was definitely not easy. In fact, it was extremely hard because of all the emotions and mental work involved in dealing with victims of Dementia. My

The Heart and Soul of Caregiving

daily motivation is the gratification that comes from being of service. I was able to make a difference in these people's lives. From a medical emergency to the solution of a small problem, a caregiver brings relief, aid and comfort.

This family was truly a gift for my loved ones and myself. Because of our job, my husband was able to finish his Nursing Degree. Our three boys were able to enroll in good schools. By helping their family, they in turn helped ours to have a brighter future.

Losing Ann

After three years of battling with Alzheimer's, Ann fought no more. She was my first patient who passed. It was a very painful experience and it was a big loss for me. The passing was kind of surreal because I was with her every day, for three years. I held her hand, embraced her and stayed by her side, for most of her waking hours in those years. A huge part of me was lost. She had become a part of my daily life. Suddenly,

Jacqueline Jennifer

one morning, she was gone. In a way, I was glad that she was finally resting in peace. Alzheimer's is a sad disease.

I grieved for Peter who lost his other precious half. I saw with my own eyes what "the other half" truly means in a marriage. They were one together. Without his beloved, Peter was never whole. I sensed that void in him. He was so sad and torn.

Paul

Paul was a very loving son with a very huge heart. He named his boat after his mother, which I found very sweet. I wish that one of my sons might do the same for me one day.

The sons of Ann grieved in their own way for their mother. Paul cried a lot.

We cried together, bawling like kids. It was so heartbreaking and so sad. But I thought, this is the family's first

Jacqueline Jennifer

loss and I needed to be strong for them. I had to keep it together because they needed me to be there. I am the caregiver.

Peter cried like a baby. Somewhere, in between his sobs, I felt his denial. He didn't want to accept his wife's passing. All the sons came daily to check on their dad and talked about their fun memories with their mom. Peter would always break down and cry. They cried together each time.

The sons sat me down in the kitchen one night and asked me to stay with their dad and continue to care for him. Of course, I gladly accepted. I still got to keep my job. Most importantly, Peter would not be alone. He had become a father to me.

It was kind of awkward during the

The Heart and Soul of Caregiving

first few days. The circumstances had changed. Without Ann, there was really nothing much to do around the house. I didn't actually know how to deal with Peter. He was always independent and I never wanted him to feel that I was there to take care of him, although that was what I did.

I asked if I could accompany him on his walks outside and he graciously agreed. He was always a gentleman, so I didn't really know if he was just being extra polite. I told him that the walks would make me feel happy and comforted, because I miss Ann.

He would just cry out of the blue and then keep quiet. I let him be. I just gave him a hug once in a while. He would always say, "You're a great lady."

Days passed and I was running

out of chores. I scrubbed the floor, rearranged and organized the cupboards, cleaned the bathrooms, the carpets, the kitchen and I cooked. I wanted to do something worthwhile. I wasn't comfortable getting paid and not doing anything. That's just me.

Maybe I was also trying to help myself, because I was grieving inside. I really didn't know how to deal with it. Ann's passing was a significant loss.

The family's feelings of grief, most especially Peter's, were more important than mine. I was focused on how I could help them move on through the process. I know that the first step of grief is *Acceptance*. Peter cried most of the time, for many days after Ann passed.

After a few weeks, the sons decided to start their vegetable garden. It was

The Heart and Soul of Caregiving

one of their lifelong family traditions. Each year, all of them come together and grow vegetables in the backyard. Peter would watch his boys work together, as they had always done. I know it made him so happy. That time, I offered to help by uprooting the weeds. It was actually fun and it gave me something to do. Peter appreciated it very much.

One day, while I was working outside, he called me in. I thought it was almost time for lunch. I went inside and prepared his food. Then he asked me to check on Ann. He wanted Ann to join him for lunch.

I was taken aback and seriously concerned. I didn't know how to react and I think I just froze. I didn't want to remind him that Ann had passed away.

Jacqueline Jennifer

It would break his heart all over again. I wasn't sure what was going on with him. Was he consciously in denial? Or actually in denial? So I told him that I would go check on Ann. I left him in the dining room.

I went in their bedroom, thinking, "What was I doing there?" Would I play pretend with Peter? Do I play along or should I tell him the truth?

After a few moments, I went back to the dining room. When I saw Peter, I didn't have the heart to tell him that Ann was gone. I just blurted out from nowhere that Ann was asleep and couldn't join him for lunch.

After that, I called all his sons and told them about the new situation. One of them told me that it's better to be truthful about it, even if it hurts. I just

The Heart and Soul of Caregiving

thought it was easier said than done.

That night, Paul was scheduled to come. He greeted his father and sat by his side. They had their usual conversation, without any mention of Ann. When Paul was about to leave, Peter asked him to check on his mother and say goodnight to her before leaving.

Paul had the same look as I had that day! He froze, stared at his dad then looked at me. After a few seconds he did exactly the same thing as I did. He went in the bedroom, waited for a few seconds, then went back to his dad and told him that his mother was resting. Then he left, baffled.

The whole situation was so new to all of us that it was difficult to know exactly the right things to do or say. I don't think there's a comprehensive manual

Jacqueline Jennifer

for that, because each person is different. Each family dynamic is different.

I felt that my role as a caregiver was to be there for them. I didn't have to fix the situation; I just had to be there.

Hot Chocolate, Apple Pie and a Dose of Insulin

My husband Joonee began his nursing school studies right before I started my caregiving job. He graduated around the time that Ann passed away. He would often help me out with Ann on days when I needed a day off. He loved how Ann would always greet him with a warm smile each morning. She never gave him a hard time getting dressed. Ann was very cooperative with him most of the time, if not always. They had a routine each morning and at bedtime. Before he took care of Peter's needs, he would help me tuck Ann into bed every night.

Joonee and Peter had a routine as well. It all started when Peter got too shaky to give himself a shot of insulin. I saw him struggle one morning and I had to offer my help. I was so afraid he might give himself too much medication. It was a big concern and I told my husband about it. Since then, even if I was there for Ann, I gradually introduced my help to Peter. I didn't want him to feel that I was taking his independence away and I didn't want to cripple him either. Sometimes too much help is not good. I felt he needed to keep his daily routine, to stay productive and mentally active. I only offered to assist him when needed help.

The Heart and Soul of Caregiving

That day, Joonee offered to help Peter with his medications. Almost every night since then, patient and caregiver followed a specific routine. Joonee would come to pick me up around 8:30 P.M. After Ann would kiss Peter goodnight, Joonee would tuck her into bed. Then he would prepare Peter's medication, warm up some hot chocolate and slice a piece of Dutch Apple Pie. He would bring it to the living room, where Peter usually sat by the fire, enjoying a book and a cup of tea. Joonee began to massage Peter's knees with heat lotion.

They would usually discuss how their days had gone. Peter would sometimes crack a joke or two that he had read in the Reader's Digest earlier in the day. Joonee would share his highs and lows and worries. The older man had a very calming effect on him. His greatest worries, of school, his finals and the board exam, seemed to vanish each time Peter assured him that things were going to be all right. And it always did! Peter never offered anything to fix it, but the way he assured him not to worry, gave him a sense of comfort. My husband totally believed that everything would be okay, because again, Peter was always right!

Peter and I

After Ann passed, it took a while before Peter and I could adjust to the situation. We were both thrown out of balance when we lost Ann. He had a routine all to himself, but my daily activities had revolved around Ann. I struggled a little at the beginning. I didn't want to hover all over Peter because I knew he loved his space. I am always conscious about respecting what other people want most, especially in their own homes. I always

Jacqueline Jennifer

made sure that I drew a line and respected the boundaries between my patient and myself. I love them, but a caregiver needs to be professional about the relationship.

In the mornings when I would come in around 9 A.M., I would start the laundry and fix his bed. Around that time, he is usually in the kitchen preparing breakfast. That was one of the most difficult parts of the day, because he would make breakfast for two!

He cried a lot of times during the first few weeks after Ann had passed. I never believed it got any easier for him. I totally understood why he preferred to deny. Acceptance was not easy and was very painful for him. I couldn't bear the pain of watching him suffer. I offered to make breakfast for him every day. At

The Heart and Soul of Caregiving

least it spared him from having to relive the painful memories of his old routine. Ugh!

Each morning, he would get out of bed, get dressed and do some floor exercises. Then he would head straight to the couch to find his cup of coffee waiting. He would read the morning paper and smoke his pipe. I, on the other hand, would be preparing his breakfast, a soft-boiled egg, two pieces of toast, milk and a cup of cereal. After I served his breakfast, I would help him transfer his coffee and newspapers to the dining table where he would continue reading while watching the morning Fox News. He was a Republican. I would then finish the laundry, clean the bathrooms, sweep the floor, sweep the front yard, water the plants and clean up the kitchen.

Then, I would start to prepare for lunch. I always made sure that his food was well plated, because if it looks good then it will taste good! He was a Type 2 diabetic. He was concerned that he had a well-balanced diet each meal. For lunch, I served him one or two slices of toast, one glass of milk, a slice of either fish or chicken and a full serving of vegetables. I gave him ice cream or pie for dessert.

Yup, the menu doesn't look like he's got diabetes, right? I made sure that he always had the same servings of food and we never had an issue with his blood sugar. I can never forget what Peter told me, "Diabetes is the best disease, because it's the only illness that you can control. If your sugar is high, you take a shot of insulin. If it's too low, eat lots of

The Heart and Soul of Caregiving

Apple Pie!"

After lunch was downtime. I would prepare him a cup of tea before I took a break to read a book. I sat on the couch across the room from Peter with the dining room between us. We would watch the news a bit and then take a nap. Peter would usually ride his stationary bike for five minutes and then go back to his Shakespeare reading.

I love reading and would do so as often as possible. Occasionally, Peter would say "Hello" to me from across the room. Every time he did that, I would know that he wanted to chat a bit. So I would sit by his side and indulge him in a conversation.

He would often ask me what I was reading. He used to be a professor. He was a very *Shakespeare* kind of guy. I felt so embarrassed to tell him that I was reading crime and romance novels by Nora Roberts. Most literary professors do not know the pop bestseller. Peter was such a gracious person. If he judged me, I never felt it. In fact, I got him to read some of my crime novels! Actually, he read quite a few. He was a fast reader. At least after each book, we had something to talk about. Because Heaven knows, I can never relate to his Shakespeare.

  We started talking about my life and my family, and he did the same. Since then, we shared many fun conversations and he never failed to shower me with praise and positive encouragement. We developed a bond of mutual admiration and respect for each other. We just became comfortable together.

  I would often think of ways to

The Heart and Soul of Caregiving

make his days happier, unique and more creative. I tried to teach him Scrabble. He had never played the word game before, so it was hard for him to absorb all of the rules. Then he tried to teach me how to play Bridge, a very specialized game. I was not a good challenge for him. We settled on Poker. He was good at it and we played using chips. We usually played until 4 P.M. when I would start to prepare his supper.

Around that time, he would do his afternoon exercises. He would take a short walk up the canyon for ten minutes, then ride his stationary bike for another five. He would eat around 5 P.M., while watching the news and I would start to clean up the kitchen. I tried to keep him busy, so he would not be dwelling on his loss of Ann. Around 6:30 P.M.,

Jacqueline Jennifer

he would go back to his couch and read more books. I would often pile his books by his side. Sometimes Peter would read the books that his sons brought him. It kept him occupied, which was really good.

Around 7 P.M., I would build a fire in the fireplace. He loved watching the flames. I believed it was because he was recalling the good times. Peter would take his family camping all over the U.S. I enjoyed making his fire; it was a fun activity for me. I learned how to strategically position the pile of wood to make a successful fire. You learn something every day! Peter loved using the newspaper as fuel, which caused some concerns with our neighbors. There was a time when the fire department came and checked our fireplace, because a neighbor com-

The Heart and Soul of Caregiving

plained that embers were flying off the roof. Of course, Peter thought they were overreacting. He said he has been doing it for 70 years and there never had been a problem.

As soon as Peter sits by the fireplace, I would then play some classical music and prepare his pipe. He taught me how to do it. I would press the half and half tobacco into the pipe then hand it to him with his match. I loved watching him, because I sort of remembered my own grandfather whom I lost when I was thirteen years old.

Around 8 P.M., I would start to turn his bed and tidy up the house. I would read while I waited for Joonee. At the end of the day, we go home with a sense of accomplishment knowing that it was a good day for Peter. Day to day

Jacqueline Jennifer

it was like clockwork for us. We would try to do something different once in a while.

Peter's best days included time with his boys. Tuesdays presented a badminton game with Paul. Skip and his wife Laurie visited on Thursdays. Saturdays were Brian's day to fix anything in the house or the car. On Sunday Tim would visit with whomever he was dating at that time. Overall Peter had his weekly schedule full and balanced. It was perfect.

Christmas Time!

Ever since the beginning, from the very first Christmas I shared with the elderly couple, Peter gave me the task of decorating the house. It was a fun tradition for the family and I enjoyed it immensely. Unfortunately, the decorations were kept under the house, which was so creepy! I always imagined snakes or monsters would jump right at me! I would set up the lights in front of the house. I would hang them over the

Jacqueline Jennifer

plants and trees. It was so pretty. Then Paul would bring a live tree and I would decorate it. Peter would watch.

Ann used to help me out too, but she would then get antsy after a while because she wanted my attention all to herself. She was like a little kid in a way.

The next morning after the decorations had been displayed, Peter and I would make a Christmas gift list for his family and friends. Peter and Joonee would go to the VA base to shop, which they usually did every Tuesday or Thursday morning, for the different gift items. Then I would start wrapping. On Christmas morning, all the boys and their families come for a Christmas breakfast tradition of Kipper fish. Then they would exchange gifts.

The Heart and Soul of Caregiving

I rarely joined them as I spent Christmas with my own family and we usually go on a trip. When I got back, the family would lavish me with Christmas gifts.

After the holiday, I had to take down all the decorations and put them back again, in the creepy crawlspace under the house. It was not fun at all, but totally worth it! I think I even had one of the "boys" do it for me one time. I know, I should have thought of that from the very beginning.

Sunbathing Naked While Reading The Paper!

To give you an idea of proportion, Peter was about six feet two inches tall and I am barely five feet. Thankfully, I never needed to lift him. He could walk by himself with the help of a walker. He had bad knees and he knew that the walker kept him stable. Without it, he would fall. He was very careful and took his time walking from one place to another. He could step down from the sidewalk in front of the house with his walker, but there was no way he could climb the stairs with the bulky rig.

In the back, his house had a short, narrow wooden stairway going to the backyard that only had ropes that served as railings on each side. There were four uneven steps and the landing was also pitched at an uneven angle. Get the picture? Peter *never, ever* went down there since he started to use his walker. He knew better.

One morning when I arrived, Peter was finishing his breakfast. I cleaned up the kitchen and I prepared his cup of tea, which he usually enjoyed after every meal, while reading a book back on his couch. He stood up and went straight to the back door. I thought he was just trying to see if the hummingbirds ate their food in the bird feeder or to see what the

The Heart and Soul of Caregiving

rain gauge was reporting. He opened the door and I panicked. I asked him, "What are you doing?"

He replied, "I'm going down to the backyard. I need to sunbathe."

I honestly didn't know what to do or how to react. I told him it was quite impossible to go down those steps. It was so dangerous and I wouldn't be able to lift him up if he fell.

I didn't even have time to call his boys. *Peter was ready to go!* I knew his sons would let him do whatever he wanted. I knew he badly wanted to go out in the sun. It broke my heart thinking that he couldn't.

I thought about it quickly. The worst-case scenario was that we would both fall down. But it wasn't that high, just four steps. If we were careful, we

Jacqueline Jennifer

wouldn't fall that hard. The worst that could happen was we would call 911 to get us both up. I bet Peter would hate that. He never wanted us to call 911, even when Ann had episodes. He never wanted Ann to go to the hospital or the ER. He said, "We should avoid the hospital at all cost, because that's where people die." True.

So I had a plan. I told him, since there was no way to change his mind, I might as well get on the steps with him. I went down first and steadied his walker as he held on to it. We took the steps one by one. Thank God we got down safely! It was so scary. I think I was shaking more than he was! I knew the worst that could happen was he would fall on me, but since he was going down very slowly, we wouldn't fall that hard.

The Heart and Soul of Caregiving

Going up the stairs would be another challenge, but I just let him be for two hours. He found his favorite chair, stripped off his clothes and sunbathed in the nude while reading his newspaper. He was so happy and I was happy for him.

I went back into the house and called Paul. His son was on the other line, so I told his assistant that Peter was out in the garden sunbathing. I reported that I had to assist him going down the steps and not to worry in case they get notified should we have to call 911.

Paul called me right back. He was very thankful that I had helped his dad. I somehow knew that all *the boys* would feel the same and no one would blame me if anything happened. I said, "Your father is outside, under the sun, reading the newspaper, naked."

He laughed and said, "Well, I'm glad he got to do it. This might be his last. Who knows?" And indeed it was his last time sunbathing, with or without clothes.

Peter, like most seniors, had lived his life so independently that he would push his limit to do things on his own. I admired how he had lived his senior years with much passion, dignity and pride. I would never take that away from him. I knew my limitations and telling him what he should or shouldn't do was not one of them. I wasn't there 24 hours per day. He was of able mind and he knew what he was doing. I was there only to assist, not to control, not to dictate.

The Heart and Soul of Caregiving

At the time, he was 93 years old. He deserved to live his life to the very fullest. At that age, some people are sky-diving! So who am I to stop him from doing whatever he wanted?

Thanksgiving Dinner... Eat and Run!

Skip and Laurie decided to have Thanksgiving at their home in Valencia. Thanksgiving dinners have always been celebrated at Peter and Ann's house. The family thought a change of venue would create a new tradition and thoughts away from their recent loss.

Joonee and I drove Peter to Valencia. We enjoyed the lovely dinner with the family. Skip made a toast and we all took turns sharing what we were most thankful for. Throughout the meal, Peter was very quiet. After dinner, he wanted to go home right away.

His sons asked him, "What is wrong, Dad?"

Peter replied, "It isn't right to leave your mother alone in the house at Thanksgiving."

We were all speechless.

Right away, Joonee and I stood up and gathered our belongings. We drove Peter home. I thought my heart was going to break; Peter was so sad.

He was quiet on the long drive back. When we got home, I prepared his hot chocolate and gave him his insulin shot. We wished him well and said our goodnights.

The next day was a Friday. After we left, the night shift caregiver came

The Heart and Soul of Caregiving

and noticed that Peter couldn't get up. He thought it was very unusual, so he called 911. The emergency came as a shock to all of us. Peter had a stroke.

Miss Congeniality

The nurses at the hospital would never call me *Miss Congeniality*. I was probably a nightmare to them and, in retrospect, I wish I had not been so hard on them. I was Peter's advocate. His doctors felt he was dying and they asked his sons to prepare for the worst. I guess that was their job, but I knew Peter was a fighter! I would never give up on him, no matter what! I would never let him go without the chance of a good fight. So, I

Jacqueline Jennifer

rolled up my sleeves. I was determined to bring Peter back home in no time.

He could not eat, as his throat muscles were too weak to swallow. The doctors wanted to insert a G-tube, a gastrostomy tube for nourishment, but there were afraid he was not strong enough. I hoped this was just temporary.

After a few days Peter developed a fever, which carried on for several days. He was coughing too, with phlegm. One of their friends who was a nurse expressed her concern; she was afraid that Peter was already catching pneumonia.

The nurses gave Peter a Tylenol for the fever. If there was a potential of something worse, then I felt the doctor should be notified. Of course, it was not that easy to get a doctor to come.

I called my mother-in-law who is

The Heart and Soul of Caregiving

a doctor in the Philippines and I told her about the new situation. She has always been my second opinion after consulting with Peter's doctors. She too was quite concerned. I did not know anything about pneumonia then. She told me that it was an infection of the lungs and most bedridden patients develop it when there is a lack of movement. She also said that it takes forty-eight hours to culture a bacteria and Peter needed to be on antibiotics as soon as possible or he could die.

Oh, wow! I was so angry because here we are in a famous, metropolitan hospital and it is my mother-in-law, a doctor 20,000 miles away, who is the one who saved Peter's life. I called his doctor; there was no answer. I went back and forth to the empty nurse's station; maybe they were making their rounds.

Jacqueline Jennifer

I swear to God, I was frantic. I almost called 911! I seriously considered calling to report a medical emergency in a hospital. I wondered if that would be a first for them?

The next morning, I was badgering the nurses to call the doctor regarding Peter's potential for pneumonia. My mother-in-law the doctor advised me not to tell the doctors what to do; we were speculating that Peter had pneumonia. It was not something we were sure of. Secondly, there is a hierarchy in the medical world that should be respected.

The resident doctor stopped by. I told her that Peter has been coughing and his fever never went down. I recommended that he should be placed on antibiotics. The doctor actually agreed and called Peter's doctor.

The Heart and Soul of Caregiving

The sons were very anxious after I explained the situation. When his primary doctor came, I told him that Peter should be on antibiotics. He agreed and he said that he would order the prescription right away. Thank God! It was about time! The extended experience was so frustrating. The long wait for the antibiotics seemed like forever. Paul even offered to pick up the medicine, but of course it didn't work that way. Paul said, "If it was their own father, the staff would be moving much faster."

After an hour or so, the nurses gave Peter three different kinds of antibiotics because they didn't know which one would work. There wasn't enough time to culture the bacteria. They x-rayed his lungs too, and true enough, he had developed pneumonia in his left lung. I

Jacqueline Jennifer

was so upset. The big problem was that Peter couldn't go thru a G-tube operation because he was too weak! He hasn't eaten in days! It was a nightmare! Like a never-ending battle!

Don't get me wrong. I appreciate the nurses. My husband is one! I understand that things happen. Nurses and doctors are always the first to take the blame. I believe my feelings were justified. I did what I had to do because I am responsible to my patient. My job, my role and my purpose is to give care. I was Peter's advocate.

Exercise and More Exercise!

After a series of breathing treatments and respiratory therapies, Peter got better. It took a few hard weeks before the pneumonia subsided and his lungs were clear. Every day, the nurses would suction the phlegm from his chest; it is a very painful thing to watch.

His left side was affected by the stroke. Finally, he was allowed his G-tube operation and he was given food through the tube into his stomach. Finally! Now, he had energy to exercise and heal.

He could hardly speak. He was exhausted from a fierce cough and the battle of much phlegm in his lungs. At least he smiled a lot. I read him a book and talked his ears off most of the time when he was awake.

The doctors could hear us, apparently. I was not that quiet. They actually thought I was doing a great job exercising Peter's mental abilities. His physical therapist would come and I would continue my patient's exercises throughout the day.

His doctors thought Peter wasn't getting any better. His condition did not qualify him to go to rehab after he got discharged. They thought he was never getting out of the hospital alive.

Who were they to judge that? I saw

The Heart and Soul of Caregiving

with my own eyes that Peter was fighting for his life. He worked extra hard to do his exercises. It was extremely hard for him to coordinate movement. I could see the determination and frustration in his face. He was diligent with his speech therapy and after a few days he did get better.

I would wait for his doctors and ambush them in the hallway, just to show them that Peter was doing a lot better. I wanted him to go to Rehab so badly because I knew that was the only way he could get better. After annoying his doctor on a daily basis, he suggested we have Peter admitted to a different rehab facility where his uncle was the director. He thought it was worth a shot.

After several days, we got a response. Peter was accepted and we

Jacqueline Jennifer

transferred him right away, instead of sending him back home. I knew Peter wasn't going to walk anymore, but I did not want his muscles to weaken. I wanted him to get better. I felt his inner drive to recover. When he was exercising, he looked so mad. I thought he needed that anger to power a stronger will to survive. He never complained. He even exercised on his own, when I had grown too tired to count.

Getting Up... Going Home

Peter got so much better at the rehab. They got him to sit up a few minutes a day. The facility had a standing frame, which helped Peter stand up on his feet. He needed to feel his legs. We were all hopeful that he would have the strength to stand.

He was discharged after three weeks, just after Christmas. We even had our own small tree in the hospital room.

Jacqueline Jennifer

I knew that going home could be a tough one for Peter. There was an extra burden now, for all of us. It would be a huge adjustment, especially for Peter. For one, he had to sleep in a hospital bed. We needed to count all of our blessings. We got him out of the hospital! Peter was so right! We had to stay away from the hospitals, because that's where people die! We got out of there alive, a huge success!

It was a tough road ahead. Progress is one day at a time.

"I Need To Get Up!"

We got home and we set up care around the clock. My husband Joonee had passed the boards to become a Registered Nurse and he served as Peter's private nurse.

The most challenging part was learning how to feed him via the G-tube. As a caregiver, one is always learning something new.

I changed his diaper for the first time. I hadn't changed a diaper since my

Jacqueline Jennifer

last child stopped wearing them.

My husband trained us all. It took a while before we got used to the new lifestyle. I had to develop a workable system for everyone and an efficient way to log medical information. We set up a nursing station, took his vitals, administered his feeding, crushed his medications, injected his insulin shot and changed diapers. Every two hours, we had to turn him to avoid pressure sores. It was Nursing 101 overnight!

After taking care of his medical needs, I wondered how we could further care for and comfort Peter. He needed to get back to his old routine, in a new way, as he was no longer walking. He was upset most of the time, because he wanted to get up. It was totally understandable and so painful to watch. I promised my-

The Heart and Soul of Caregiving

self I wouldn't give up on Peter. I would do everything I can to help him recover, at least to the limits of his ability. His anger gave him the will to get better and stronger each day. I just let him be. I knew he needed time to process everything.

Food! Food! Food!

It was less than a week when Peter realized he wasn't eating regular food. He was getting better and stronger, which was great, but he was starting to get bored and very hungry. The doctor advised us against giving him anything by mouth. He was a high risk of pulmonary aspiration, the danger that food or other material might enter his lungs. We couldn't afford that risk after everything Peter had been through.

Jacqueline Jennifer

Every time Peter asked for food, I would change the topic or distract him. Most of the time, I would patiently explain why he cannot ingest food through his mouth. *Not just yet.* Of course, he wouldn't listen and he began to resent me. He thought we were conspiring to kill him, because we would not give him any food! This concerned me greatly and I called his son Paul who came right away.

As a rule, I never call a relative unless it is an urgent matter. First, I tried calling his doctor to ask permission to give food to my patient; I wanted to know what kind of food to give. His receptionist took a message.

Paul and I took turns. He would explain to his father why he can't eat anything through his mouth and Peter

The Heart and Soul of Caregiving

would just tell him to, "Get lost!" Peter went ballistic. The man wanted to eat and no amount of persuasion would change his mind.

Finally, the doctor called and told us that we could feed Peter *at our own risk*. He suggested puree, like baby food, thick soup or ice cream. Paul and I rattled around the kitchen, looking for something thick to give Peter. Finally we found a can of mushroom soup. We cooked and served it. After receiving his first spoonful of flavor, he looked at us and said, "See, I'm still alive! I told you!"

Paul and I looked at each other and laughed. We cried with joy for Peter. It was crazy. We got through it. I was so glad Paul was there. You can never mess with a hungry man!

Goals, Goals and More New Goals

Walking was an impossibility, but the goal to eat normally was something workable. His problem was his weakened throat muscles; he had twice failed a swallow test with video. By focusing on speech therapy and swallowing exercises, Peter could get stronger. Nutritionally, we were still feeding him through an intubated tube. Food and flavor would be for his pleasure, gratification and dignity.

Jacqueline Jennifer

I learned the proper applications and procedures. Aggressively, I started with the exercises. Every day, Peter and I would start our morning with vocal exercises, tongue, mouth and swallowing. We repeated it six to eight times a day.

We got him frozen lemon lollipops to stimulate his saliva, which actually helped with swallowing. We did everything on the book, by the book.

Then came the big day. We went to do the video swallow test. I sat with the doctor and the technician. With a camera inserted in his throat, we watched Peter swallow. He was given foods of different consistencies, from thick to thin liquids. I saw that when it came to clear liquid, Peter failed. It went down the wrong pipe and he did not even cough. The doctor said it was called silent aspiration. The

The Heart and Soul of Caregiving

stroke had been destructive.

At least he passed the test for thicker foods. His condition wasn't that bad at all. We went home and worked some more. Together, we kept at it, six to eight times a day. Peter was very cooperative and motivated.

After a few months, I rescheduled the video swallow test, and guess what? Peter passed with flying colors! It was a very proud moment for me. I cheered for him each time the food went down the right pipe! The doctor probably thought I was crazy. He just didn't know what Peter had to go through to win this victory. After everything he had lost, being able to eat normally again was a treat and a break he greatly deserved!

The doctor approved eating but he did not advise that we get rid of the G-tube.

Jacqueline Jennifer

Peter got all the nutrients he needed to recover through the G-tube, yet he still had the option to eat as he pleased. The doctor introduced the risks involved, such as aspiration pneumonia.

The boys thought the benefit was much more valuable than the risk. Eating was gratification for Peter. He deserved to enjoy his precious life. After all, he had just celebrated his 94th birthday.

We gave Peter food whenever he asked for it. This way we lessened the risk of aspiration.

I focused on fun physical exercises and brain activities. I got him an E-book and he was very appreciative of that. He started talking again. We did a lot of vocal exercises to strengthen his throat muscles and vocal chords. We played a badminton game for the bed-

The Heart and Soul of Caregiving

ridden. I got him a Skull Candy headset so that he could listen to classical music and Shakespeare audio books. He looked forward to seeing his boys and enjoyed their company at every visit. We took him to the park when the weather was nice. I maintained his busy weekly schedule. I took him to an outpatient rehab twice a week, just for the change of environment. My constant daily goal was to make his life interesting and happy.

When Ann died, Peter asked me to never leave him alone. I saw his fear and loneliness. Then and there, I promised him that I would be with him to the very end. This gave him assurance; I knew he believed me.

One day while we were sitting by his bed in front of the TV, he suddenly asked me where Ann was. I saw in his

Jacqueline Jennifer

eyes that he knew, but he needed to hear it from me. I took his hand and placed it on his heart and I told him, "This is where Ann lives." He sobbed like a child, crying out of frustration and sadness. We both cried together. He asked me again for a promise to never leave him. I said I would never leave his side. He looked scared and very sad at the same time. I laughed and said, "You'll never get rid of me, even if you wanted to!" Peter smiled and said, "Good." After a while, he fell asleep. I was happy to give him that assurance. He never asked me again after that. He knew he had me by his side no matter what.

The Doctor is In!

I have never heard of a doctor coming to visit a patient in their home. Once common, the practice is just not done anymore. My mother-in-law is a doctor in the Philippines and she makes house calls only in an emergency, in a country where there is no 911. In the U.S., doctors can no longer afford the time and money to make a house call.

I was surprised to meet this wonderful and super compassionate doc-

Jacqueline Jennifer

tor who came to see Peter in his home. This good doctor came once a month, or whenever necessary. Dr. Silva appeared at a time when we needed him the most. Due to his condition, Peter was prone to pneumonia. He began to develop the life-threatening condition every four to six months, sometimes even faster. The doctor would arrive and give him a shot of antibiotics.

Peter was well taken care of. He had someone come to draw his blood for the insulin management. A physical therapist arrived on a regular basis. Dr. Silva was impressed that Peter never had any pressure sores and his body was clean. He was happy about Peter's cognitive improvement and really took great care of him. There were a few Sundays when Dr. Silva came to see Peter when

The Heart and Soul of Caregiving

he had a fever. He even picked up his cell phone every time I called! Does anyone know of a doctor who comes even close to that? He was great doctor and I am glad we found him. Dr. Silva was part of our team and stuck by Peter to the very end.

Three long years after his stroke, Peter began to deteriorate. Throughout that time, he had been bedridden and pumped with medications of all kinds.

It all began when he became more and more agitated. At first, it was only at night. Then Peter started to become worrisome during the day. He would always say, "Help me," over and over.

The neighbors probably thought we were hurting him; there were a few times when they knocked on our door

Jacqueline Jennifer

in the middle of the night. Peter's voice got louder and louder and the only way to manage his anxiety was to give him medication to calm him down. The sedative was necessary because his blood pressure became too high whenever he got upset. It was very stressful for everyone, most especially for Peter.

His sons didn't know how to react when they heard their dad in such distress. I saw how uncomfortable and frustrated they were. Sometimes I would give Peter a massage to calm him down prior to his children's visits. I wanted them to enjoy their conversation and company.

It was a pity; many times they came to visit when their dad was dozing on and off. I asked them to come during the daytime when he was the most active and awake. I took a video of Peter playing

The Heart and Soul of Caregiving

bed-badminton and reading; I emailed it to his sons. I wanted them to see their dad happy and serene. Peter and I would call his boys and he left them a message on their voicemail. Usually, Peter was asleep whenever they called back. There was always something every day and I thank God for the opportunity to make a difference in this family's life.

I began this journey to feed my family, pay our bills and educate my children. I never imagined it would turn out to be a life-changing experience.

My brother once told me, "In life, never chase the money. Chase your heart and its desires. Money will follow." It is very true, especially in this case. I focused on taking care of my patients, making them important and the main

Jacqueline Jennifer

purpose of my daily life. In return, their family took care of mine. My kids were able to study in good schools. My husband finished his nursing degree with which he was able to secure a good job in the middle of an economic recession.

When my husband graduated from nursing school, Peter and my other patient Eileen attended his graduation party. I was so honored and humbled that they took the time to drive all the way to be a part of our special celebration. Peter's son Skip came as well. It was so awesome. It was one of the most significant events of our lives. Joonee got a job right away at a prominent nursing facility, just a stone's throw from our home.

When Peter had his stroke, Joonee was offered a job at the best rehab cen-

The Heart and Soul of Caregiving

ter in Beverly Hills, but he chose to turn it down. He knew Peter needed him. To help the loss of income, he took a job as a Utilization Review Nurse, which he could easily do since all he needed was a computer. The pay was not much, but he knew Peter mattered to him, and to us, even more. After all, he was like a father to Joonee in so many ways. Peter made a huge impact on his life.

That dreadful phone call came from the night nurse one morning around 5 A.M. Peter was not well and his blood pressure was very high. His breathing was labored. We were afraid that he might get another stroke.

Joonee and I got up and called Dr. Silva who came around 6 A.M. We had arrived a half an hour earlier. Peter was wheezing badly. Joonee immediately sat him up and administered a breathing treatment. Peter tried to cough up his phlegm with difficulty. It all happened very quickly. Peter's vitals were very unstable. We coached him to breathe in and out. *Calm down. Do not panic.*

The doctor came and gave him a shot of antibiotics. There was nothing else he could do. He instructed us to continue our efforts and then he left.

Peter wasn't getting any better. His phlegm was so thick; he had a hard time coughing it out. His blood pressure began to decline quickly. While again on the phone with the doctor, Silva instructed us to call 911. We stayed by Peter's side. Joonee was assuring him that help was coming and that he should calm down, relax and breathe in and out.

The Heart and Soul of Caregiving

I called all the sons. I had a very bad feeling about it. I never thought a decline could happen so fast. I was not prepared for it. Of course, we all knew that day was coming, but Peter and I had an agreement that he would live up to a hundred years. I even said, "Let's make it a 105." It was all happening too soon.

The Promises that We Keep

At the ER, most of the family was present.

Paul was in Colorado and his signal was very poor; no one could reach him. He had driven there, so it would take a long time for him to head back; I was worried that he might be too upset to drive. I called his girlfriend and she didn't know how to tell Paul either. We asked Skip to be the one to break the news to his brother.

Jacqueline Jennifer

Peter had another aneurism and it was a big one. It affected most of his brain. If he lived, he would have been dependent on machines and he would not be able to talk or function normally. He would be far worse than his previous condition. The doctors needed their decision then and there.

This time, I didn't yet know what was going on. I was just anxious to get Peter out of the hospital. I was ready to face whatever challenges were headed our way and I knew it was going to be more difficult than ever before. But Peter was a fighter. I would fight for him if he couldn't fight for himself. If he were in a coma, I would blast his ears with Shakespeare audiobooks until he woke up! I would talk to him and scold him and motivate him to fight.

The Heart and Soul of Caregiving

The next day, Skip, Brian and Tim were all there with Laurie, Linda and Peter, Skip's eldest son. One of them informed me that Paul needed to be contacted because a family decision had to be made.

That was it. I knew it was the day. I snapped out of myself and focused on Peter's sons. They loved their father so much. He had been their rock all of their lives and I needed to stand by them and be strong. I didn't even know how to help them. I wished I could make it all better for all of them. I knew I did all I could for Peter, but somehow I always felt I could have done more. Of course, I knew better than to go down that route.

Paul gave his okay to his brothers. He didn't want them to wait for him.

A little later, I called Paul and we

cried so hard on the phone. I once told him that losing your parents make you feel like an orphan. No matter how old you get, as long as you have a mother or a father, you will always remain a child to them. Once they're gone, you are on your own. I am sure this doesn't hold true for everyone. That's just how I felt when I lost my father at a young age. I felt I had to grow up fast. I told Paul to drive safely and to pull over if he wasn't feeling okay.

The social worker came and asked me if I had a particular religion. I said I was a Catholic.

She asked me if I wanted a priest to bless Peter. I told her that the family is not particularly religious and it wasn't my place to decide. I promised

The Heart and Soul of Caregiving

her that I would mention it to the sons, which I did when they all came back from lunch. Skip in particular asked me what I thought. I took it as an opportunity to speak my mind. I always hoped for Peter to be blessed by a priest ever since he had a stroke. We talked about it a couple of times, but I never acted upon it. Peter was not a religious man, but he always had the patience to listen. Every Sunday, for the last six years, his friends Sam and Theresa came to visit and they would study the Bible. He prayed with them and read the Bible when asked. Peter once told me he was baptized a Catholic in England. He went to a Catholic school in Australia and he encouraged all his grandkids to study in Catholic schools because he believed in the quality of the Catholic Education.

Jacqueline Jennifer

Being a Catholic myself, I told Skip that having a priest pray for Peter would be a very good idea. Besides, I didn't think it would hurt. He had asked me, so I don't think I was crossing a line.

The doctors called the family together for a meeting in a conference room. I stayed in the ICU with Peter. Skip came back and asked me to join them. It was very humbling and I was deeply honored. While we were all sitting around the table, the doctors began to discuss the gravity of Peter's condition. It meant the family must decide if they were ready to pull the plug. Paul had given his approval and the family was in unison. It was the best thing to do for their dad.

The doctors got their permission from each family member. As they start-

The Heart and Soul of Caregiving

ed to discuss the medical procedure and what will happen next, Skip stopped them and asked me what I thought. He asked in such a way that I realized my opinion really mattered. My relationship with the family was valued. I was touched, and taken aback as well. Naturally, I agreed. This was the best thing to do for my patient. There was no doubt about it. I didn't want him to live a miserable life. It would be unfair and selfish to keep him alive with machines.

The social worker, also in attendance, asked the family again if they wanted a religious blessing. Skip said, "Yes." She asked what denomination would they prefer. Skip asked me again and I replied, "A Catholic Priest." It made a huge difference for me, knowing that Peter will be given his last rights. I

Jacqueline Jennifer

felt he was going to be okay.

The priest came and talked to the sons before going into Peter's ICU room. True to his tradition, he was very nice and respectful. When he learned that Brian went to a different church, something I was never aware of, he asked the family if they preferred to gave their dad a generic blessing. They all agreed. For me, any blessing is good enough. We all went in and gathered around Peter. This was the first time I saw the family bow their heads and pray together. It was a very solemn moment. I was grateful to have been a part of it.

The prayer and blessing were nice, brief and truly special. After the priest left, each family member said their goodbye to the patriarch of their family.

A nurse arrived and told them that

The Heart and Soul of Caregiving

she was going to unplug the machines.

For me, it felt so sudden, like they were in a hurry. I never understood the haste. Was somebody else going to use the room? I just kept it to myself. I didn't want to make a scene. It just didn't sit well with me. Of course, I was in so much distress and pain. An angry reaction was my defense.

Everyone decided to leave. They could not bear to watch their dad die. This is probably one of the most painful experiences a person has to go through in life. I would do the same if I were in their shoes. I loved this family so much that I would do anything to protect them.

As they left one by one, Skip asked me if I was going as well. I told them I would stay with their dad for a while. I'm sure they felt better knowing I was there beside Peter.

In truth, I stayed because I was keeping my promise to my patient: to be there beside him until the very end, to hold his hand, and to never, ever leave his side until he was gone. I felt so blessed to have the opportunity to keep my special promise.

The nurse came into the room and began to unplug the loud machines and turn off the beeping monitors. Reality began to kick in. I began to cry. The sum of all of our hard work, hopes and fears were coming to an end. Peter was dying.

The nurse comforted me. She let me know that her team was closely monitoring Peter's heart from their station. She pledged to come and tell me herself as soon as he had passed. The situation was inevitable. Peter's time on earth was

The Heart and Soul of Caregiving

coming to an end.

After the nurse left, the room was now quiet and still. Peter's eyes were slightly open and I felt he could see me. Peter was in a coma and I knew he did not feel any discomfort or pain.

I held his hands and I thanked him for all of our years together. He was so good to me. I thanked him for his kindness and for being so gracious. I thanked him for being so appreciative and loving. I told him how grateful I was to have had him in my life.

I promised him that I would always be here for his boys. I told him I loved him very much. He was a great man, I said. I will greatly miss his very calm way of comforting and reassuring me that the challenges in life will always turn out all right. I told him how happy I

Jacqueline Jennifer

was that my children had the opportunity to meet such a gentle and strong soul. He was a very special part of our lives.

I held his hands as I spoke to him. I like to believe that he could hear me. I even called out to Ann and told her that she would soon be with her husband once again. In many ways, I felt that she had never left his side. I told them both that my family and I would miss them very much.

This moment of goodbye was so surreal, but I did not want to let the experience pass me by. I felt every minute that was left. I wanted to cherish it. I squeezed Peter's hand and said, "You know I keep my promises."

Slowly, his pink cheeks began to pale and turn to white. I literally saw his blood stop flowing and I felt it in the

The Heart and Soul of Caregiving

hands I was holding. It was an amazing and beautiful experience for me. I looked at my watch. The time was 3:30 P.M.

The nurse came into the room. I told her what she already knew.

I saw Skip in the lobby. The rest of the family had already left. I told Skip his dad was gone and we cried and we wept. He called his brothers to let them know.

Skip drove us home because at that time I had no car. As we walked to the parking lot, I told him how everything had worked out just fine. I felt his pain and shock; it had all happened so suddenly.

When he had the stroke the first time, everyone thought Peter would never make it home from the hospital.

Jacqueline Jennifer

I reminded Skip that it had been just a matter of time before something would have happened again. We were so lucky to have prolonged his life for three more years. Paul called it *borrowed time*. The fact that Peter did not suffer and died so quickly was a great way to go. He was in a coma when they pulled the plug. He didn't feel a thing. Peter had a peaceful death. Skip realized I was right. We all did our best and his sons provided their dad with the very best care.

Skip felt a little bit better; already he was missing his dad. He wasn't prepared, but I don't think anyone can ever be. There would be much more grief and pain to be felt. He had just lost his father, a great man, whom he had loved and respected all his life.

A Caregiver

A client and friend once told me that my job as a caregiver sucks. I asked him, "Why?" He said, "Because people die." True, but what makes it worthwhile is knowing that I made a difference in their lives. I made their days better with comfort and love. I was there to make them laugh when they were sad or hold their hand when they were scared.

The joy of caregiving is the little things that make a big difference, one

Jacqueline Jennifer

moment at a time. That is what caregiving is all about.

These rewards are far greater than the pain of losing them at the end of their journey. Life is short, but the opportunities to help and to touch other people's lives are endless. This is the heart and soul of a caregiver.

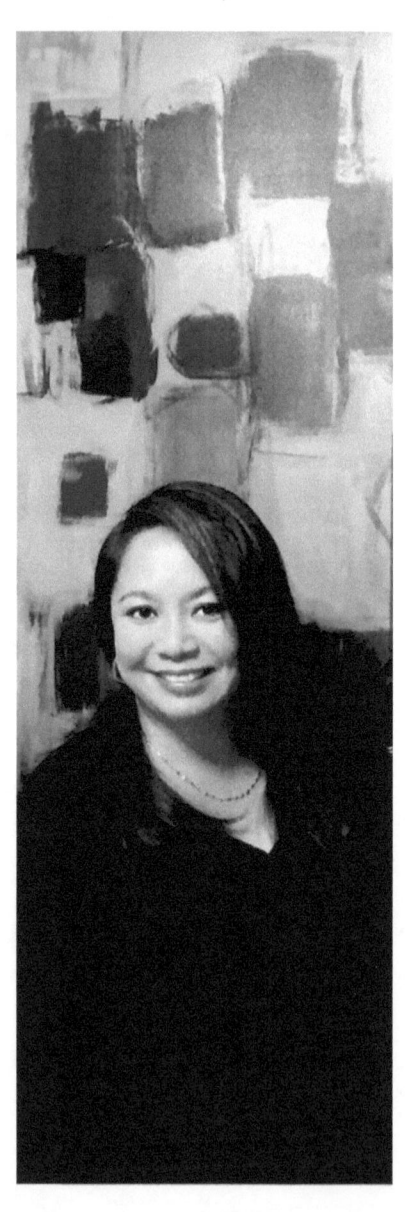

About the Author

Jacqueline Jennifer has found her passion as a caregiver. Today, she is the hands-on president of a small but dedicated firm devoted to giving care and solace to those in need.

Born and raised in Manila, Jacqueline grew up in a big, loving family of seven. Soon after college, at the age of 21, she married her husband and became a proud mother to three amazing boys.

Jacqueline brings a wealth of necessary skills to the caregiving profession. She and her husband have ventured into a diverse variety of businesses. From

Jacqueline Jennifer

construction management to fashion design to trading, they have even owned and managed a commercial fishing boat. Facing the challenges of raising a family at an early age, Jacqueline and her husband wanted to succeed. They set their sights on America.

While he earned his nursing school degree, Jacqueline and her husband supported each other with a series of odd jobs, each with a promise of advancement and success. One job in particular began to resonate. Jacqueline cared for an elderly patient, mending a broken hip. At once, everything fell into place. Jacqueline found her calling and passion in life. Quite naturally, she took caregiving to a higher level. She made it her profession.

The Heart and Soul of Caregiving

Jacqueline's good work was noticed and demand exceeded supply. With the help of family and the support of her clients, Jacqueline Jennifer established her own agency. With years of experience and expertise, she developed an amazing team of caregivers who share her passion and dedication to make a difference in the lives of her clients.

CONTACT THE AUTHOR AT:
JOONJACKBOOKS@GMAIL.COM

The Heart and Soul of Caregiving

www.ingramcontent.com/pod-product-compliance
Lightning Source LLC
Chambersburg PA
CBHW030936180526
45163CB00002B/589